MEDICAL LIMERICKS II

by

William J. Stone, MD

MEDICAL LIMERICKS II

©2013 by William J. Stone
All rights reserved. Printed in United States of America. No portion of this publication may be reproduced in any manner without written permission of the author.

ISBN-13: 978-1491205785
ISBN-10: 1491205784

Library of Congress Control Number 2013905988
CreateSpace, North Charleston, S.C., USA

Book cover design and desktop publishing by Mary Margaret Alsobrook Peel. Ms. Peel is a Medical Illustrator and currently serves as the Chief of Medical Media at the Department of Veterans Affairs Medical Center where she directs illustration, graphic design, photography, and other visual support for medical, patient and staff teaching programs.

Dedicated to

*The Men and Women
Who have served
in our Armed Forces,
Our Veterans.*

FISTULA FIRST

Save veins named cephalic and basilic.

For access they are not thrombophilic.

Into an abyss or vortex

Hurl catheters and Goretex,

And life will be almost idyllic.

Note: Arteriovenous fistulas using native vessels can last for more than 20 years and are less prone to clot or become infected. Both PTFE (Goretex) fistulas and, particularly, central venous catheters are much more likely to clot or to become infected.

Ref: Clin J Am Soc Nephrol 2007; 2:786-800.

THIS WORMY WORLD

A round worm named Strongyloides

Is tiny next to A. lumbricoides.

It lives in our guts,

Makes tracks on our butts,

And goes wild when it eats STEROIDES.

Note: Glucocorticoids are transforming growth factors for this roundworm, greatly increasing the number of worms and changing non-invasive larvae to the type that can bore through the bowel wall. Normal hosts can carry the parasite in small numbers for years, only to become seriously ill when treated with glucocorticoids for any reason. Bacteremia with intestinal flora is a common presentation. No geographic area is immune.

Refs: Rev Infect Dis 1989; 11:755-767; Sem Resp Infect 1990; 5:58-64.

OCD[1] NEPHROLOGY

Arcane renal diseases from A to Z:
Names like Drash, Gordon, Hartnup, Fabry,
Liddle, Zellweger and Bartter,
You must study them harder,
Or you'll blow that outrageous Boards fee.

Note: Older doctors, who write board examinations, are often enamored by eponyms. These names can be used to describe syndromes, diseases, physical findings, and other aspects of the practice of medicine.

1 Obsessive Compulsive Disorder

SIAADH[2]

Bed-wetting kept him up all night.

A doctor sought to ease his plight.

The enuresis to lessen

He was given desmopressin,

But his sodium then dropped out of sight.

Note: Desmopressin is not a good treatment for enuresis, unless the patient is carefully taught fluid restriction and followed for the development of hyponatremia.

2 The syndrome of the inappropriate administration of ADH – a true story.

LESS IS LESS

A number of nephrons is sown ya.

When enough, they won't have to clone ya.

If you're born with too few,

Kidney damage will accrue,

Called oligo-mega-nephronia.

Note: When there are fewer nephrons because of disease, surgery, or birth defects, the remaining glomeruli tend to hypertrophy. This leads to premature senescence and progressive loss of kidney function.

THE DEMON GODDESS PODAGRA[3]

Gout is a disease most obdurate

Caused by crystals of sodium urate.

Arthritis and tophi to fix

Keep the serum level under six.

Joint symptoms will often ameliorate.

Note: Gout has afflicted mankind for centuries and always will. We each have an inactivating mutation in the gene for urate oxidase. As long as the serum urate stays under 6 mg/dl we will not accumulate crystals of sodium urate in our joints and tissues. Neither will we have gouty arthritis or tophi. Those that have clinical gout can be successfully managed with allopurinol or febuxostat, but must realize that it is a life-long problem. The goal of therapy is a consistent serum urate level under 6 mg/dl.

Refs: Am J Med 1996; 100 (suppl 2A): 46s-52s; NEJM 2005; 353: 2450-61.

[3] Podagra is a character in a Roman play by Lucian, who lived in Greece in the 2nd century AD.

PERICARDIAL CONSTRICTION

Massive edema went up to his thighs.

To Nashville for heart transplant he flies.

Cards wanted him quickly listed,

But our team only persisted.

Cardiac echo gave us quite a surprise.

It wasn't that his heart was spent.

A strange shadow around it was bent.

To the OR he travelled.

The problem was unraveled.

An unchained heart his Christmas present.

Note: Diagnosis of constrictive pericarditis can be difficult, particularly in separating it from a restrictive cardiomyopathy. The clue here was a mononucleosis-like illness, which took this vigorous athlete to a state of being unable to walk a few feet within 6 months. Surgical correction is not always easy.

Ref: NEJM 2000; 343:106.

THE CHAMP (OF DISEASE)

Tiny molecules swim in the sea

Of human fluids like plasma and pee.

Reactive oxygen species,

The list never ceases,

But the greatest is NF kappa B!

Note: NF-kB is a family of pleiotropic transcription factors that integrate an intricate network of extracellular pathways. Hundreds of genes related to immunity, inflammation, apoptosis, cell proliferation, and cell differentiation are regulated.

Ref: J Am Soc Nephrol 2010; 21:1254-62.

CHOLESTEROL EMBOLISM

Chest pain struck an old man from Paris.

"It's angina", said Doctor Harris.

In the cath lab he froze,

He came back with blue toes,

And livedo reticularis.

All of his muscles started aching.

Kidneys and GI tract were quaking.

Eosinophilia appeared,

And more complement was cleared,

As his BP new records was breaking.

Note: Atheroembolism is a significant complication of atherosclerosis. It varies from tiny emboli of cholesterol crystals to pieces of plaque occluding larger arteries. Often misdiagnosed, it is usually caused by arterial catheters.

Ref: Am J Med 1996; 100: 524-529.

THE COCCI BELT

If you happen to have HIV

Or other immune deficiency

There lives a tiny pest

In the desert Southwest

That you should avoid assiduously.

Note: Coccidiomycosis is an endemic and serious fungal infection of the U.S. Southwest. Arthrospores are released into the air by wind, earthquakes, construction of buildings and excavation. It can cause anything from a mild illness to pneumonia and meningitis. Tourism, with return to non-endemic areas before becoming ill, can lead to misdiagnosis. Immunosuppression can activate latent infection.

Refs: Mayo Clin Proc 2008; 83: 343-49; J Infect Dis 1995; 171: 1672-5.

THE AMERICAN WAY OF DEATH

(or Why our Dialysis Mortality is so High)

Although the U.S. population is varied,

And an array of genes is carried,

It certainly is no myth

Our "rights" endow us with

A dialysis catheter to be buried.

Note: We are spending an enormous quantity of our healthcare dollars on the last few months of life in our elderly population. ICD/pacemakers and hemodialysis catheters should be carefully considered before being placed in an elderly patient with a shortened life expectancy.

Ref: Clin J Am Soc Nephrol 2012; 7:2049-57.

UNILATERAL RENAL ATROPHY WITH COMPENSATORY HYPERTROPHY

A scan the radiologist visualizes,

Showing kidneys of two different sizes.

The first was oh so small,

It was nothing at all.

The other was large and won prizes.

Note: Unilateral renal atrophy, because of birth defects or disease, causes compensatory enlargement of the opposite kidney (providing it is normal). The earlier in life this occurs, the greater the effect. Even middle-aged renal transplant donors wind up with two-thirds, not one-half, of prior renal function.

PANHYPOPITUITARISM

It struck him while watching The Preakness,

Nausea, lethargy and weakness.

He felt cold in warm air,

Lost all his body hair,

Plus libido, reflexes and sleekness.

Note: This is partial or complete loss of anterior pituitary hormone secretion. It is usually permanent. In older adults the non-specific symptoms may be dismissed by the patient or the physician as due to aging. Treatment regimens must be tailored to the patient.

Ref: Lancet 1998; 352:127-34.

"BELIEVE IT OR NOT"

A strange new treatment came to us,

Which our pig friends so kindly grew us.

It's for ulcerative colitis

And regional enteritis,

Using the roundworm Trichuris suis.

Note: Exposure to helminths is thought to prevent or ameliorate inflammatory bowel disease. Trichuris suis was used in this study of Crohn's disease and showed a positive result.

Ref: Gut 2005; 54: 87-90 and 6-8.

BEER POTOMANIA

His caloric intake was only beer:

Six packs and kegs for year after year.

We fed him hot dogs

And bacon from hogs.

Hyponatremia did disappear.

Note: Two six-packs of beer contain over 4 liters of water and virtually no residual solute (Na, K, Cl, nitrogen). Solute is needed to excrete water. Minimum urine osmolality is about 50 mosm/l, so 200 mosm would be needed to excrete the 4 liters.

Ref: Am J Kidney Dis 1998; 31: 1028-1031.

THE NEGLECTED VITAL SIGN

Blood pressure, pulse, respirations are great;

Even O2 sat. and temp. are first rate.

But in patients with nephrosis,

Heart failure, or cirrhosis

Would you please obtain a daily weight!

Note: In the management of edematous patients undergoing diuretic therapy, there is nothing so key to a shortened hospital stay as accompanying fluid restriction. Daily weights are an important parameter to follow. Diuresis begins at 3-4 liters of urine output per day. The patient should be weighed standing, if at all possible. Fluid should be restricted to one liter per day.

ADRENAL CRISIS

Anorexia, weight loss and asthenia

Progress toward hypovolemia.

Vitality nearly ceases

As skin pigment increases.

Could it be hypocortisolemia?

Addison figured out this disease,

Which brings patients down to their knees.

Hyponatremic and they vomit.

Potassium rises like a comet.

Florinef/prednisone will put them at ease.

Note: Adrenal insufficiency is often confused with more common disorders. I encountered an elderly man who had been put on a clinical research study of platelet turnover. A low salt diet was part of the study. He rapidly deteriorated, but the reason was unclear until I came along. He was Addisonian.

Ref: Am J Med 2010; 123:409-13.

PICA

Laundry starch, toilet paper, river bank clay,

Celery, carrots or chalk day-by-day,

They eat ice by the pound,

Whatever crunchy can be found.

Iron will cure their humiliation right away.

Note: Pica is often missed in an admission history and physical examination. It is caused by iron deficiency in many cases and may cease when the patient is iron-replete. "Crunchy" edibles seem to be the common denominator.

Ref: JAMA 1976; 235:2765.

PEG-YLATED

Many diseases assailed an old man;

As death approached he gathered his clan.

PEG tubes to the rescue.

They're as common as fescue.

Don't put them in just because you can.

Note: The pun refers to polyethylene glycolation of protein drugs to prolong their half-lives, as in erythropoietin. Lengthening the life of a cancer-ridden patient by tube feedings requires careful thought and consultation with the patient and family. PEG (percutaneous endoscopic gastrostomy) tubes can be very helpful in certain settings, but they do not prolong life in advanced dementia.

Ref: Arch Intern Med 2003; 163:1351-53.

AVE SAINT THOMAS

One of West Nashville's most imposing sights

Great patients, Nutty Buddies, chopper flights

Johnsons, Campbells, Doctor Rods

How they taught us in the pods

Will Eric Sumner please turn off the lights.

Note: This was a sentimental tribute to the Catholic hospital which helped train Vanderbilt residents and medical students over many years. The excellent attending physicians and last Chief Medical Resident are cited when the relationship was discontinued. Nutty Buddies were available 24/7.

"CELL"-ulitis

It afflicts half of all Nashvillians

And Americans by the millions.

Their turn signals don't work

They drive me berserk,

And they run stop lights by the zillions.

Note: I wrote this after almost being hit by an SUV running a red light. The driver was talking on his cell phone as he proceeded merrily along.

AN EMERGING GREAT DISEASE

Lymphoma is one of those diseases

That behaves any way it pleases.

With treatments that are new

We can conquer it too,

If our diligence never ceases.

Note: A great disease has 3 characteristics:

- A. It is sneaky and has many presentations that can throw you off.
- B. It is potentially fatal.
- C. It is treatable!

TOBACCO IS NOT COOL

There was an old man from Sewanee

Who had a cancer in his kidney.

There was more in his bladder.

His lungs were even sadder.

It's because he smoked like a chimney.

Note: Tobacco use is slowly declining in our population, but the misery it has left behind is mind-numbing. I never cease to stress, in a serious tone, the many harmful side effects of smoking to addicted patients. Finally, I urge them that now is the time to quit.

PNH

You don't have to be a New Yorker

To mutate genes that sound like a porker.

Cytopenias and more,

Blood transfusions galore,

Excess clotting is the real corker.

Note: The disease is paroxysmal nocturnal hemoglobinuria (PNH). All patients have mutations in an X-linked gene called PIGA which lead to dysfunction of certain proteins anchored to the cell membrane. Complications include hemolysis, smooth muscle dystonia, and thrombosis.

Ref: Ann Intern Med 2008; 148: 587-95.

CURVULARIA KERATITIS

When you're seven, the future is dim.

Hurt in your yard? The chances are slim.

Throw a ball in a tree,

One of its branches breaks free.

A rare fungus comes down with the limb.

Note: The trauma from the branch transmitted a fungal keratitis to the boy. In Mandel's text of infectious diseases in discussing this entity, the following statement is made: An antecedent vegetable injury may have occurred.

WHEN FIBER ISN'T GOOD FOR YOU

There's a serum protein called TTR.

When mutated, it caused amyloid S50R.

Our patient had cardiomyopathy,

Diarrhea and neuropathy.

Diagnosis was worth a gold star.

Note: Hereditary amyloidoses are most often related to mutations in transthyretin (TTR). They present as some combination of peripheral neuropathy (similar to diabetic), cardiomyopathy and/or nephropathy. Treatment is supportive, but it is important to make the diagnosis. Amyloids are polymeric proteins formed into fibers in humans, which injure normal tissue. Not all are caused by plasma cell dyscrasias or mutations.

Refs: Mayo Clin Proc 1992; 67:428-440; Blood 2009; 114: 4957-59.

HEAD AND NECK CANCER

Can't swallow, mouth hurts, covered with drool,

Depressed because he feels like a fool.

With appetite nearly ceasing,

Belt size ever decreasing,

Will someone tell kids that tobacco isn't cool.

Note: It is the 6th leading cancer world-wide. It usually is a squamous cell carcinoma. Tobacco, human papilloma virus, and alcoholism are risk factors. Men in their 60's and 70's are most affected. The 5-year survival rate is 40-50%.

Ref: J Clin Oncol 2006; 24: 2137-50.

A SALUTE TO EDWIN NEWMAN[4]

"Appreciate" murmurs, how about hear?

It's a diagram not a "cartoon," I fear.

"Endorses" chest pain or has?

Users of "you know" I razz.

"Basically" is the useless word of the year.

Note: There is a growing use of inappropriate jargon in both written notes and oral patient presentations.

[4] Edwin Newman is the author of "Strictly Speaking. Will America Be the Death of English?"

OGLALA SIOUX

Plains Indian I could see at a glance,

Chest scars from many a Sun Dance.

Short of breath, wounded heart,

Fluid balance off the chart,

Diuresis his spirit will enhance.

Note: This Native American made a living selling tee shirts about Sioux history at fairs and flea markets. He had participated in Sun Dances as a young man. This involves the peoples of the Plains Nations. Dancers are ritually pierced in the ceremony. The patient was older and suffering from heart failure.

LYME DISEASE IN TENNESSEE?

A nursing student had arthralgias

Fatigue, weakness, and myalgias.

To the internet she went.

Lyme Disease was her bent,

And caused her doctors many cephalgias.

Leukocytes and complement were low.

Fever and azotemia were seen also.

Her renal tissue was sounded.

Immune complexes abounded.

Lupus therapy has restored her glow.

Note: Renal biopsy showed Stage IV lupus nephritis. She is now more than 10 years out on minimal immunosuppression. It is controversial whether Lyme Disease exists in Tennessee. Current goals in lupus nephritis are to achieve complete remission quickly and to prevent relapses.

Ref: Kidney Int Suppl 2012; 2:221-232.

YOU CAN LEAD A HORSE TO WATER
BUT YOU CAN'T MAKE HIM DRINK (HYPODIPSIA)

High sodium since his aneurysm got a band.

Urine osmolality well over a thousand.

Too much salt in his diet.

Tap water, will he try it?

When he does, everything is grand.

Note: Healthy elderly men have a reduced sense of thirst after a water deprivation test. The thirst center in the hypothalamus is also near that for vasopressin release and may have been affected by the banding of the cerebral aneurysm.

Ref: NEJM 1984; 311: 753-59; Am J Med 1982; 73: 354-356.

OYSTERITIS

Vibrios do multiply in warm seas

From Florida all the way to Belize.

In months that have an "R"

Shellfish are safer by far.

In spring and summer they carry disease.

Note: The old saying about months with an "R" is not strictly true. September and October are still dangerous times in the Gulf of Mexico. Vibrio vulnificus infection is almost exclusively seen in raw oyster eaters, often with cirrhosis. Of 422 infections with V. vulnificus between 1988 and 1996 reported to the CDC, 45% were wound infections and 43% were primary septicemia. The septic patients were 86% male and 96% ate raw oysters. The mortality rate was 61%.

Ref: J Infect Dis 1998; 178:752-759.

INTRADUCTAL BREAST CARCINOMA

A woman was rapidly dying[5],

But her tumor was oh so benign.

Like a bear in the woods,

Breast cancer has the goods

To gobble liver without even trying.

Note: In this patient the supposedly less malignant intraductal breast cancer was growing up the hepatic sinusoids. Liver failure resulted from loss of normal liver cells. It was quickly fatal.

[5] Of fulminant hepatic failure

WHY I LIKE AN ALL-ELECTRIC HOME[6]

This colorless, odorless gas

Binds to hemoglobin quite fast.

Victims have such a headache,

Get dizzy, stomachs quake.

Diagnosis requires a doctor first class.

Note: Carbon monoxide results from incomplete oxidation of carbon-based fuels. Faulty gas appliances, vehicle exhaust, and wood or charcoal fires are among the many causes. If you use such in living spaces, you will need a carbon monoxide detector. Mount it at the ceiling. Carbon monoxide is lighter than air.

Ref: NEJM 2002; 347: 1057-67.

[6] No carbon monoxide

INTERSTITIAL NEPHRITIS

When the renal interstitium is inflamed,

A plethora of medications can be blamed:

Sulfas, NSAIDs, penicillins,

Quinolones and cephalosporins.

Stopping drugs this syndrome has tamed.

Note: Although there are much less common other causes, a variety of medications can be implicated in most patients. Findings include an increasing serum creatinine, hematuria, leukocyturia, and modest proteinuria. Some patients require transient dialysis.

Refs: J Am Soc Nephrol 1998; 9:506-151; Clin Gastroenterol Hepatol 2006; 4:597-604.

CROHN'S DISEASE

IBD grabs your gut like a crab.

Of course, they've been working in the lab.

To cure fistulas, iritis,

Pyodermas and arthritis,

You can be treated with infliximab.

Note: Infliximab is a chimeric monoclonal antibody which targets TNF-alpha. It has been used in moderate-to-severe Crohn's disease since 1998. Results have been promising.

Ref: NEJM 2010; 362:1383-95.

BOWEL PREP

If bowel cleansing you contemplate,

Make sure not to use any phosphate,

Such as enemas by Fleet,

And Visicol please delete,

Or the kidneys you may soon ablate.

Note: Phosphate is an under appreciated toxin and should only be used briefly in phosphate-depleted patients. It causes both acute and chronic nephropathy and arterial calcification.

Ref: J Am Soc Nephrol 2005:16:3389

WHAT'S IN A NAME ?

First under the Neisserian umbrella,

Next known by the genus Branhamella.

Species catarrhalis has stuck,

But you're just out of luck,

If you're not aware, it's now Moraxella.

Note: Moraxella is an aerobic, gram negative coccobacillus which causes otitis, sinusitis, pneumonitis and endocarditis.

Ref: South Med J 1999; 92: 1071-74.

SUITE METHEMOGLOBINEMIA

Whether bronch, TEE or EGD,

Benzocaine spray's used quite liberally.

Deep cyanosis, brown blood,

Doctors panic, call a code.

Methylene blue is preferred therapy.

Note: One of our faculty had a TEE at another hospital. He turned blue, was intubated, and received a Swan-Ganz catheter while fully awake. Methemoglobin levels were high when eventually measured. Benzocaine usage is not quantifiable and can be dangerous.

Ref: Medicine 2004; 83: 265-273.

TRAIN WRECK

Shipped comatose from another VA,

Renal transplant, all organs gone astray.

Digits bulging with tophi.

The BUN was sky high,

And aortic valve chewed by MRSA.

Note: This patient had MRSA endocarditis, which carries a high mortality in renal transplant recipients (44%). There is a 170-fold risk compared to the general population. Tophaceous gout was another problem in this patient taking cyclosporine. It is not seen during tacrolimus therapy.

Refs: J Am Soc Nephrol 2000; 11: 974-79; Transpl Int 2005; 18: 690-96.

HEPATOERYTHROPOIESIS

EPO's an important drug in our quiver.

In renal failure it's a key health-giver.

But this may all be passé.

New agents are on the way

That cause EPO production by the liver.

Note: The reasons for inadequate erythropoietin (EPO) production in ESRD are poorly understood. Hypoxia-inducible factors (HIFs) are being targeted for pharmacologic intervention. An orally active prolyl-hydroxylase inhibitor to stabilize HIF worked in 12 hemodialysis patients, 6 of whom were surgically anephric. EPO levels increased 31-fold in nephric and 15-fold in anephric subjects. This enhanced EPO production in anephrics is presumed to be of hepatic origin.

Ref: J Am Soc Nephrol 2010; 21:2151-56.

GINSENG LUNG

Many people after ginseng do lust.

Fifty pounds a year he dug from the earth's crust,

Roots overhead he did toss.

Came cough, dyspnea, weight loss.

Sporothrix he'd inhaled with the dust.

Note: Ginseng is a valuable commodity prized as an aphrodisiac. There is an art to finding this root in the woods. It is often sold on the black market. This patient cleaned loose soil off the harvest by shaking the plants over his head. He inhaled Sporothrix in the process, leading to cavitary lung disease. Diagnosis was made by culture of bronchoscopic washings. Itraconazole therapy for 18 months resolved the lesions.

Refs: Tennessee Medicine 1999; 92: 306; Clin Infect Dis 1995; 21:981-85.

WARFARIN BLUES

There is a drug known as warfarin.

A panacea it never has been;

Because drug interactions

And co-morbid reactions

Bring on bleeding much to our chagrin.

Note: Warfarin complications are frequent. Development of atrial fibrillation should not result in its use in every patient. Bleeding into the CNS, GI tract, and retroperitoneum are especially dangerous.

Refs: Ann Intern Med 2003; 138: 831-38; ibid 1994; 121: 676-83: Am J Med 2007; 120: 700-705.

DERMATITIS HIEMALIS (WINTER ITCH)

When cold weather arrives to stay,

Comes pruritus that won't go away.

On wet skin post-lather

Lots of lanolin you slather.

Flaky hide will new life display.

Note: The older that you get, the more dry skin is a problem. Applying a lanolin-based lotion over damp skin can ease the symptoms. It prevents evaporative losses. Bathing should also be limited to once a day.

EMPHYSEMA ON CHEST FILMS

Shrugged shoulders, wide intercostal spaces,

Bullous change normal lung tissue replaces.

Blood vessels are not there,

Too much retrosternal air,

Flattened diaphragms down at the bases.

Note: Criteria include: 1) flattening of the diaphragm on the PA film; 2) irregular radiolucency; 3) increased retrosternal air space on the lateral film; and 4) flattening of the diaphragm on the lateral film. The "shrugged shoulders" sign is due to increased lung volume and is accompanied by increased clavicular angles.

Ref: Diagnosis of Diseases of the Chest (4th edition), 1999, volume III, pp. 2204-2209, Fraser and Paré, eds.

THIAZOLIDINEDIONES

A group of drugs ending in "glitazone"

Works on PPAR gamma, it's newly known.

Increased function of ENAC

Compels salt/water to flow back,

Making patients more edema-prone.

Note: These drugs are ligands for peroxisome proliferator-activated receptors (PPARs). Rosiglitazone is a specific ligand for the gamma isoform and is used to treat diabetes mellitius. However, it also stimulates ENAC to reabsorb sodium and cause edema in 5% of subjects. ENAC is a sodium channel in the renal collecting tubule.

Ref: Nat Med 2005; 11: 861-67.

LPR

Persistent cough, lots of throat clearing,

Local soreness and dysphagia appearing.

It's intermittent, not chronic.

Voice breaks, is dysphonic.

Patient and doctor some cancer are fearing.

If gastric juice makes it to laryngeal,

It's called reflux, laryngopharyngeal.

Symptoms occur upright,

Unlike GERD that's at night.

Six months of PPI will be needed to heal.

Note: Patients are often misdiagnosed as sinusitis. Incorrect referral to ENT specialists results. They usually have no esophagitis or its primary symptom, heartburn. Their reflux occurs during the day. The upper esophageal sphincter is dysfunctional, rather than the lower one as in GERD.

Ref: Otolaryngol Head Neck Surg 2002; 127: 32-35

TOO MUCH ENAC

There's a syndrome named after Grant Liddle.

Its hypokalemic hypertension was quite a riddle.

Aldo and renin were low.

Spironolactone's no go.

Triamterene kept serum K right in the middle.

Note: This is a genetic disease where there is a gain of function mutation in the epithelial sodium channel (ENAC) of the collecting tubule, causing hyperabsorption of sodium and excess potassium secretion. It mimics primary hyperaldosteronism, except plasma aldosterone levels are suppressed. Amiloride and triamterene block ENAC and are adjuncts to a salt-restricted diet.

Ref: Kidney Int 1998; 53:18-24.

"DIRTY" URINE

Is it "dirty" blood aswarm with staphylococci,

Or "dirty" CSF teeming with cryptococci?

Let's keep our language so clean

That it reveals what is seen

With beauty like the daisy named ox-eye.

Note: Another piece of inexact jargon that has crept into the medical language of today. I might accept "dirty urine" as a feature of a cystocolonic fistula.

CC: "IT'S MY TRANSAMIN, DOC."

An inflamed pancreas is pancreatitis,

Infected lungs we term pneumonitis.

But there is not a doubt

That I can't figure out

What organ's ailing in transaminitis.

Note: Once we discover where the "transamin" is, we can work on preventing ESTD (end-stage transamin disease). Transaminitis is an incorrect term which should be abandoned, but is in common usage by residents. It is incorrectly applied to elevations in the serum ALT and AST, when other liver tests are normal. Rhabdomyolysis can be misdiagnosed as "transaminitis".

NORMOCEPHALIC, ATRAUMATIC

The French Revolution blew a gasket.

Then King Louis' head fell in a basket.

It was normocephalic,

But not atraumatic,

Headless Louis wound up in a casket.

Note: These useless terms appear in most written physical examinations and need to be deleted.

KEEPING REGULAR

When a presenter says "regular rate,"

Dr. Bart Campbell starts to agitate.

It's rhythm that's regular,

Or it can be irregular,

While rate is speed, e.g. one twenty eight.

Note: This feature of many physical examinations is often shortened to RRR, "regular rate and rhythm." I was guilty in the distant past of using it. However, rate is speed and cannot be designated as regular.

Ref: JAMA 1989; 262:3338.

CARTOONS

Comical drawings which something lampoons,

Often with words rising up in balloons.

Grand Rounds slides slowly drag by.

This term to them does not apply.

Power Point diagrams are not cartoons.

Note: For Gen Xers: if you want to see the world's best cartoons, check out the "New Yorker" magazine.

WHERE THE SUN DON'T SHINE

They are usually covered by apparel,

Sometimes smelly and far from sterile.

Stop being timid and look.

Get back to ways you forsook.

You have abandoned them at your peril.

They're an important part of the physical.

Why we don't do them to me is quizzical.

We abhor the "Genital,"

And even more the "Rectal."

When omitted, their lack can be critical.

Note: I have observed in recent years that there is a reluctance among house officers to perform genital/rectal exams. Diagnoses that are missed include anal cancer, fissures, ulcers, prostate cancer, BPH, hydrocele, testicular masses, Fournier's gangrene, penile lesions and more.

LUNG ABSCESS

Fever, cough, anorexia, malaise,

He's been sick for over fifty-nine days.

Thick sputum is grayish-green.

It smells just like a latrine

From booze, bad teeth, and neglectful ways.

Antibiotics and drainage will commence.

Also critical is the patient's adherence.

Improvement will be slow,

For anaerobes are the foe.

Most of all the doctor with need patience.

Note: This is an indolent process developing over weeks. Aspiration leads to necrosis of lung parenchyma in a dependent segment. A density with an air-fluid level is seen on chest films. Multiple bacteria, especially anaerobes, are involved. Clindamycin and ampicillin sulbactam are often given until the process is cleared.

Ref: Curr Infect Dis Rep 2000, 2:238-244.

NITROFURANTOIN LUNG

Paraplegic having chronic UTI's,

Macrobid to cut infections down to size.

Dyspneic to the nth degree,

Infiltrates seen on chest CT.

Prophylaxis almost led to his demise.

Note: This drug is sold under many brand names. Chronic use can lead to pulmonary toxicity of a severe nature. It is mainly seen in elderly women who present with respiratory symptoms after being treated for a year or more to suppress recurrent urinary infections. Ground-glass opacities are seen on chest imaging. Cessation of the drug may lead to improvement.

Ref: Mayo Clin Proc 2005; 80:1298-1302.

HYMENOPTERA

In my back yard while serenely mowing,

Came small bombers not made by Boeing.

Yellow jackets are most fierce.

Thrice my hide they did pierce.

Maybe this chore I should be forgoing.

Note: Allergic reactions to insect stings are common and can be serious, even fatal. Immunotherapy can prevent anaphylaxis in the majority of those affected.

Ref: NEJM 1994; 331:523-27.

DRUG-INDUCED HYPERKALEMIA

Aldactone, salt substitutes, heparin,

NSAIDs, tacrolimus, cyclosporine,

Amiloride, triamterene,

Trimethoprim, pentamidine

ACE inhibitors and ARB's to begin.

Note: Non-steroidal anti-inflammatory drugs (NSAIDS), spironolactone, KCl-containing salt substitutes, eplerenone, heparins, ACE inhibitors, angiotensin receptor blockers, other K salts, beta blockers, labetalol, antibiotics and COX-2 inhibitors can be implicated in causing hyperkalemia. Chronic kidney disease is a co-conspirator.

Ref: Am J Med 2000; 109:307-314.

TREATING HYPERNATREMIA

Twice their weight in kilos gives the rate

Of oral water or D-five they'll tolerate.

To get the number of hours

Ere they wilt like dry flowers,

Twice the delta sodium will be just great.

Note: These are formulas that I developed using a body water of 0.6 l/kg. The rate in ml/hr is twice the patient's weight (kg), so that the serum Na does not fall faster than 0.5 mEq/liter/hour. The delta sodium is the amount that you want to decrease that value in mEq/liter. These volumes are added to maintenance fluids. Serum sodium should be monitored during treatment. In obese patients use ideal body weight.

TRIAD OF EXCELLENCE

Address patient problems with intelligence.

Attack your daily tasks with due diligence.

Rare cases do us enthrall,

But remember most of all

To treat each soul with awesome reverence.

REFUGEE

He's a "Lost Boy," a native African.

Visited friends in Uganda, not Sudan.

Prophylaxis he did not take.

Came back with fever, bad headache.

Mefloquine turned him into a new man.

Note: This was astutely diagnosed as falciparum malaria at the Siloam Clinic by Dr. David Gregory. The patient recovered nicely on antimalarial therapy. With airline travel able to bring people from the world-over to the U.S. in 24 hours, we need to widen our differential diagnoses.

Ref: Ann Intern Med 2013; 158: 456-68.

ONE OF PATTON'S FINEST

Drop attacks at eighty went unimpeded.

Slow rate, a pacer was badly needed.

Had a clot within his heart.

"Cards" a skillful plan did chart.

The result our best hopes far exceeded.

Note: This patient was a sergeant who led a motorized howitzer crew in Patton's Third Army (WWII). At age 89 years, he has lived 7 more years despite his ischemic cardiac disease and chronic GI bleeding from an unresectable colonic adenoma. "Cards" refers to a cardiology consultant.

DIRE COMPLICATION

From another hospital where he's been seen,

"Perirectal abscess" was all they could glean

His genitalia were sore,

The perineum even more.

Necrotic skin revealed Fournier's gangrene.

Note: This is a rapid necrotizing cellulitis of the anogenital region, which is due to a mixed aerobic/anaerobic infection. It is a surgical emergency. The surgeons did a great job with this patient. A perforation of the urogenital or lower GI tract is often etiologic.

Ref: J Urol 2008; 180:944-48.

THE CLIENTS

Our patients think of us as giants.

We insist on their full compliance.

What started doctors to say

A term I treat with dismay.

Only "Hair Club for Men" has clients.

Note: The doctor-patient relationship should be much more personal. Despite our busy schedules, time and energy must be allotted to maintaining it. To me, calling patients "clients" denigrates it.

IT'S ONLY FOR VEHICLES

Comatose, seizures, in a dire strait,

Gap acidosis, little urine, but wait.

Many kayak-shaped crystals

Spoke louder than two pistols.

Antifreeze had put him into this state.

Note: Urine microscopy showed the characteristic crystals (calcium oxalate monohydrate) of ethylene glycol poisoning. He recovered both renal and mental function following a course of hemodialysis and psychiatric therapy of depression, which had led to a suicide attempt.

Ref: Clin J Am Soc Nephrol 2008; 3:208-225.

CAN YOU URINATE AND CHEW GUM AT THE SAME TIME?

The urologists have a clever test.

The causes of bloody urine are addressed.

Three bottles in which you piddle:

Early, late, and in the middle.

Hand-eye-bladder coordination is assessed.

Note: The so-called 3 glass or 3 tube test has been used for decades. More red cells early indicates a lower tract source (urethra, prostate) and late is from the bladder trigone. Equal red cells in all 3 containers is from the upper tracts, including kidneys and ureters, or from diffuse bladder involvement. However, this is not a great test and is a challenge to female patients in particular.

.

CLOSTRIDIUM SEPTICUM

No one knew his right colon hid a mass.

We were preoccupied with all the gas.

Subq emphysema

Blossomed out of edema.

Clostridial sepsis did him in quite fast.

Note: Bacteremia with this organism often heralds an undiagnosed colon cancer, esp. cecal. It is the most common cause of spontaneous, nontraumatic gas gangrene. Illness is usually fulminant, causing death within 24 hours. The initial amount of subcutaneous gas may be trivial, but it soon takes over the clinical findings.

Refs: Rev Infect Dis 1990; 12:286-296; NEJM 2000; 343: 1615.

NEW DISEASE

Home dialysis, active worker, new hip pain.

All images negative that we could obtain.

Then his femoral neck broke.

A strange diagnosis was evoked.

Beta 2 M amyloid on Congo red stain.

Note: It wasn't simple, but this Nashville VA patient led to the discovery of a new kind of amyloidosis in 1985. It was a polymer of normal beta-2 microglobulin, which accumulates in plasma levels 30-50 times normal in dialysis patients and leads to skeletal amyloid deposits. This is an amyloid that weakens bone, leading to fractures, and which deposits in joints and the spinal column.

Ref: Semin Dial 2006; 19:105-109.

OLIGURIA POST - UNINEPHRECTOMY

One kidney, rapidly rising creatinine.

Stones in the past, little urine was seen.

No hydro on ultrasound.

Urology we had to hound.

Retrograde got things flowing by 9:15.

Note: Renal US is not perfect. You will occasionally see obstructive uropathy with a normal US. Patients with one kidney and an increasing serum creatinine have obstruction until proven otherwise. This patient had 2 prior episodes, yet urology balked due to the "normal" US.

Ref: BMJ 1990; 301: 944-46.

PSEUDO-NEPHROTOXICITY

What can falsely raise the creatinine?

Azole antifungals, cimetidine,

States of ketoacidosis,

Bactrim for pneumocystosis,

Cephalosporins and eating creatine.

Note: This is marked by an elevation in the serum creatinine, but the BUN stays roughly the same. Cimetidine, azole antifungals, and trimethoprim block creatinine secretion in the proximal tubule. Cephalosporins and acetoacetate interfere with the assay of creatinine. Ingestion of creatine by exercise enthusiasts (e.g. body builders) enhances creatinine production.

INCREASED BUN TO SERUM CREATININE RATIO

Figuring this out is not just symbolic,

Prerenal states such as caused by colic.

Rule out internal bleeding,

Too high a protein feeding,

And glucocorticoids can make one catabolic.

Note: GI, retroperitoneal, or soft tissue hemorrhage is turned into urea, as are high nitrogen diets including enteral and parenteral nutrition. Urinary obstruction, with stagnant urine sitting next to epithelium, is also a cause. Glucocorticoids, in a dose-dependent manner, increase protein catabolism. Pre-renal states can only triple the BUN above baseline due to a concentrated urine and enhanced proximal urea reabsorption.

Ref: Kidney Int 2002; 62:2223-29.

PLAIN-SPOKEN

"To be honest" is a hackneyed phrase,

Suggesting dishonesty on previous days.

"Like" and "actually" are unneeded,

And "basically" should be weeded.

"To be perfectly honest" an even worse cliche.

Note: These are commonly heard in medical presentations, waste time, and need deletion.

VALACYCLOVIR NEUROTOXICITY

Zoster struck him, to Derm. Clinic he went.

ESRD; lowered dose was not sent.

Excess Valtrex he was taking,

So confused, limbs were shaking.

Two dialyses, he was over the torment.

Note: Extensive dose reduction of valacyclovir, acyclovir and related drugs must be done in patients with advanced CKD or who are on dialysis. The main metabolite, CMMG, is neurotoxic. Confusion, disturbances of consciousness and hallucinations are most common.

Refs: Eur J Neurol 2009; 16: 457-460; J Antimicrob Chemother 2006; 57:945-949.

CRYSTAL CLEAR

Altered mentation and myoclonic jerks,

Was it meningitis or herpes that lurks?

Antibiotics, quite robust,

Yellow urine turned to "pus".

Acyclovir crystals had gummed up the works.

Note: A column of white material was pushing clear yellow urine down the Foley catheter drainage tube. There were no white cells in the spun urine, only massive, fine, needle-shaped crystals of acyclovir. Parenteral acyclovir had been given to treat possible herpes encephalitis in an HIV/AIDS patient on HAART.

Ref: Arch Pathol Lab Med 2002; 126: 753-54; Am J Kidney Dis 1993; 22: 611-15.

CONSULT

Don't use "consider" or "may" in your text,

Or "what's reasonable" when making your recs.

Excess verbiage is a waste.

Simply cut to the chase.

Please briefly tell me what to do next.

Note: I believe that the consult note in the medical record does not need to recapitulate what is already known about the patient. It should focus on additional facts, suggestions about further studies, and changes in therapy, for starters. It should be brief and to the point.

HYPERCALCEMIA

Nausea, vomiting, constipation,

Confusion, GFR alteration,

Polyuria, weight loss,

Even yelling at the boss,

The cause needs a quick investigation.

Hyperparathyroidism, carcinomas,

Paget's disease, myeloma, lymphomas

Vitamin D, milk-alkali,

Rare causes also roll by,

And sarcoid plus other granulomas.

Note: This is a classic presentation that has a myriad of confusing signs and symptoms. Nuances can help in the differential diagnosis being narrowed. Acronyms for it abound. Malignancy-associated hypercalcemia is chiefly mediated by PTHrp, RANKL and MIP-1.

Ref: Leukemia Lymphoma 2004; 45:397-400; J Am Soc Nephrol 2008; 19:672-75.

EXOPHTHALMOS

His right eye protruding, was it glaucoma?

Cervical node biopsy showed carcinoma.

There was a lot of discharge;

Orbital muscles were large.

Pseudo-Graves would not be a misnomer.

Note: This patient's proptosis was unilateral and mimicked Graves' ophthalmopathy. Images of the orbit showed enlarged musculature. Biopsy revealed invasion by the disseminated carcinoma. This is an unusual site of metastases. Palliative radiation is being given.

Ref: Case Rep Ophthalmol 2011; 2:360-66.

PSEUDOTUMOR MEDIASTINII

Fatigue, cough, his appetite slowed,

High calcium, a big mediastinal node.

Sure that it was some cancer,

We had a much better answer.

Sarcoid was what node biopsy showed.

Note: Mediastinoscopy with lymph node biopsy led to the diagnosis of sarcoidosis. In this illness 40% have hypercalciuria, 11% hypercalcemia and 10% calcium stones. Overproduction of calcitriol by the granulomatous tissue is responsible. Glucocorticoid therapy is helpful, but must be managed carefully.

Ref: Ann Intern Med 2012; 156: ITC5-1 to ITC5-16.

MYELOMA KIDNEY

He came billed as obstructive uropathy

And had uremic encephalopathy.

Light chains in serum amassed,

Urine filled with long casts.

Renal biopsy showed cast nephropathy.

Note: The BUN was over 200 mg/dl, serum creatinine was 23 mg/dl, and renal US was normal. The diagnosis of myeloma was suggested by refractile casts, some of which crossed the entire field at 500x magnification. When the serum immunofixation electrophoresis returned, a thick band of monoclonal light chains was seen. Renal disease is a not uncommon presentation of myeloma. Diagnosis of MM requires having it in your differential of undiagnosed renal insufficiency.

Ref: J Am Soc Nephrol 2012; 23: 1777-81.

EXTREME NEUTROPHILIA

Half are infections like pneumonitis.

Lymphoma and CML also can bite us.

G-CSF, SIRS syndrome,

Hemorrhage and prednisone,

Don't omit pseudomembranous colitis.

Note: When greater than 12,500 neutrophils per microliter are reported in peripheral blood, there is a broad differential diagnosis. In one study of 100 patients only 48% had an infection. However, an increasing infectious cause is pseudomembranous colitis due to Clostridium difficile.

Refs: Am J Med 1998; 104:12-16 and Am J Med 2003; 115:543-546

DRUG-INDUCED NEUTROPENIA

Beta-lactams, dapsone, macrolides,

Antivirals, seizure meds., sulfonamides,

Immunosuppressants, NSAIDs,

Psychotropics for our heads,

Sulfonylureas, ACEIs, and antithyroids.

Note: This is a moderately common issue in patients not receiving chemotherapy. One of the newest causes is cocaine contaminated with levamisole.

Refs: Ann Intern Med 2007; 146:657-665; Am J Clin Pathol 2010; 133:466-72.

EL BAZO GRANDE[7]

In his abdomen a mass did remain.

It was huge, shaped like the land of Spain.

Not lymphomatosis,

'Twas myelofibrosis.

We decided to call it the Splain.

Note: Chronic idiopathic myelofibrosis occurs in elderly patients and presents with marrow fibrosis, an abnormal peripheral blood smear and striking splenomegaly. The most frequent causes of death relate to marrow failure, transformation to AML, and portal hypertension.

Ref: NEJM 2000; 342:1255-65.

[7] Massive splenomegaly in Español.

MOLLITIES OSSIUM

Eight months of back pain, growing fatigue.

Compression fracture heightened the intrigue.

There was pancytopenia,

Ten grams of globulinemia.

His chiropractor was clearly out of his league.

Note: Multiple myeloma was first described by Macintyre and Solly in the mid-1800's. It represents ten percent of hematologic malignancies and, unlike this patient, can be quite sneaky. It is thought to be incurable. New therapies are under investigation.

Ref: Clin Biochem Rev 2009; 30:93-103.

HIGH ON LIFE

If a drug injector you've chosen to be,

You'll wind up cirrhotic from hepatitis C.

Rare glomerulonephritis

Or cryo. vasculitis,

But hepatoma your final misery.

Note: The highest odds ratios for having HCV are: injection drug use - 49.6, blood transfusion (esp. pre-1990)-10.9, and sex with an injection drug user – 6.3. Everything else is 2.9 or less. By 2007 HCV had superseded HIV as a cause of death in the United States. The deaths disproportionately occur in middle-aged persons. It is the leading cause of hepatocellular carcinoma.

Refs: Ann Intern Med 2012; 156:271-278; ibid 2013; 158:329-337.

OSTEITIS FIBROSA CYSTICA

Stones and fractures from osteopenia,

Neuro changes due to hypercalcemia.

Some go to the OR;

Others get Sensipar,

No longer feeling crushed by La Nina.

Note: Primary hyperparathyroidism is often asymptomatic; but can present as lithiasis, a compression fracture, mental status changes, or renal disease, among others. Fuller Albright was the investigator who led the way in the 1930's to defining this disease and its therapy.

Refs: Clin J Am Soc Nephrol 2009; 4:1541-46; NEJM 2000; 343:1863-75.

HEPCIDIN

There's a new molecule called hepcidin,

An inhibitor of ferroportin.

It keeps iron in storage,

Causes iron absorption blockage,

And results in anemia creeping in.

Note: Hepcidin does not kill the liver, but is a normal gene product secreted by the liver. It rhymes with "sid-in not side-in". Called the "master regulator" of iron homeostasis, it is a small peptide (25 amino acids) which was discovered in 2000. Inflammation increases hepcidin levels and decreases the availability of iron for red blood cell production, i.e. anemia of chronic disease. Two patients in Boston with liver tumors had severe microcytic anemia which was unresponsive to IV iron. The tumors were overproducing hepcidin. Surgical resection cured these anemias. Mutations in the gene for hepcidin, HAMP, result in juvenile hemochromatosis. Hepcidin levels are also high in kidney failure. A hepcidin antagonist could be useful in treating the anemia of ESRD.

Refs.: Clin J Am Soc Nephrol 2009; 4:1384-87.

VASCULITIS

Cocaine user with little self-control,

On and off drugs, but they're taking a toll.

White blood cells recurrently low,

Purpuric lesions began to show,

Because his "coke" was cut with levamisole.

Note: When you see a cutaneous vasculitis, keep this one in mind. The cocaine epidemic continues. Levamisole is an antihelminthic with immunomodulatory properties that is now only used by veterinarians. It is found in 70% of seized cocaine in the U.S. Apparently it is thought to enhance the "high" of cocaine. Complications of this adulterant were first reported in 2009. They include a cutaneous vasculitis (often of the ear lobes), a thrombotic vasculopathy, and neutropenia/agranulocytosis (69%). There is a 27% rate of recurrence on reexposure to adulterated cocaine. The syndrome usually wanes in a short time. Whether G-CSF or GM-CSF should be used is controversial. ANCA may be seen.

Refs.: Clin Toxicol 2012; 50:231-241; Curr Opin Hematol 2012; 19:27-31.

A BOTTLE OF POISON

He said a friend gave him some "mountain dew".

Confused, lethargic, and gait was askew.

Anion gap hit thirty three;

Creatinine rising steadily.

Urine microscopy again came through.

Note: The urine exam with my office microscope demonstrated the canoe-shaped crystals of calcium oxalate monohydrate. These are invariably missed by routine laboratory urinalysis. Almost all of the pitfalls of ethylene/diethylene glycol poisoning were illustrated in this patient. He was first triaged to mental health, laboratory results were delayed and misinterpreted (high anion gap with no osmolar gap), and nephrology was not initially consulted despite an increasing serum creatinine. The anion gap was over 30, which indicated a glycol, methanol or lactic acidosis. The glycol had already been metabolized (no osmolar gap). He was not diagnosed or hemodialyzed until the crystals were seen, which may be too late to save kidney function (oxalosis). However, in this instance he did recover at least a third of normal renal function. The cause of this poisoning is being investigated.

Ref.: Semin Dial 1994; 7:338.

NEW FRONTERS IN NON-COMPLIANCE

Asked his doctor about a swallowed gold crown.

Belly film the radiologist did astound.

Twenty six dense objects there,

Chewing binders he did forswear.

Lanthanum pills cut in pieces he had downed.

Note: Lanthanum carbonate is a recent addition to the phosphate binder armamentarium. These agents are used to prevent complications of hyperphosphatemia in ESRD patients; e.g. vascular calcification. Lanthanum is a heavy metal ("rare earth") next to barium in the Periodic Table (element 57, atomic weight 139). It is radio-dense. To be effective it must be chewed before ingestion. Swallowing this large tablet whole or cutting it in pieces (6 in this case) will not do the job. Patients do not like the idea of having to chew these pills. Finally, the gold crown from one of his teeth was not seen on the film!

Ref.: NEJM 2010; 362:1312.

COKE ADDICTION

She drank two to three gallons of coke per day.

Suddenly dropped dead, her life in disarray.

Pathologist blamed caffeine,

Or low K it might have been.

I'd bet brain swelling caused her to pass away.

Note: This 30 year-old mother in New Zealand died of a cardiac arrest as she was getting her 8 children ready for school. She had been ill for months with low food intake. She smoked 1.5 packs of cigarettes per day. The local coroner attributed her death to a "heart attack" due to hypokalemia and caffeine from the Coca-Cola. The above intake of soft drink had been going on for months. Of course, one could not rule out premature coronary artery disease from heavy smoking. However, I believe this is another example of ingesting large volumes of dilute fluids with inadequate dietary solute to enable excretion of H2O. Severe hyponatremia and cerebral edema can cause sudden death.

Refs.: Am J Kidney Dis 1998; 31:1028-31; NEJM 2005: 352;1550-56.

T-TUBE METABOLIC ACIDOSIS

Biliary T-tube causing volume depletion.

Acute kidney failure as a complication.

Serum chloride was 116,

And bicarb's down to 14.

Bile has a high bicarb concentration.

Note: This patient was discharged from a surgical service postcholecystectomy with a T-tube draining to an external bag. Since then he has had 2 admissions to the medical service for hyperchloremic acidosis (anion gap 11), volume depletion, and acute kidney injury. Inadequate replacement led to this result. A little known fact is that selective removal (as here) of biliary and/or pancreatic secretions (net base of 50-70 meq/liter) will cause this syndrome unless adequate volume and bicarbonate supplements are given. Thus it is on the differential diagnosis list of normal anion gap metabolic acidosis, along with all the 3 types of renal tubular acidosis, diarrhea, replacement of bladder with bowel segments, NH_4Cl use, and massive saline infusion.

Ref.: Dig Dis Sci 1987; 32:1033.

SPUN OUT

There's a new fitness boom called spinning,

A coach yelling while you're madly cycling.

But a woman with sickle trait

Cycled into a dire strait

Because all of her muscles were lysing.

Note: Rhabdomyolysis can be seen in the context of heavy exercise in normal individuals, particularly if they eschew adequate training beforehand. Marathons, triathlons, military settings, and various sports have contributed cases. Sometimes hereditary muscle diseases are uncovered. Sickle trait was first reported as a cause in a series of 4 African American recruits undergoing basic combat training in El Paso, TX (altitude 4,000 feet). All died of shock, acute renal failure, and hyperkalemia from rhabdomyolysis. Sickled muscle vasculature was seen at autopsy. All had been previously healthy. Many cases have been reported since then in non-military persons. How to handle this difficulty has been very controversial.

Ref: NEJM 1987; 317:781-787.

IV DRUG ABUSE ENDOCARDITIS

IV drugs kept him strung out and broke,

But this illness sure wasn't a joke.

First the mitral valve blew.

Then the aortic went too.

Enterococci came in with the coke.

After new valves they thought he was home free,

But a lump enlarged behind his right knee.

The answer was exotic.

An aneurysm mycotic

Lurked in his popliteal artery.

Note: This is one of the most severe complications of IVDA. Left-sided endocarditis is far worse than that on the right in this setting. The rate in IVDA's is 2-5% per year. Staph. aureus is the most common organism. The tricuspid valve is infected in 60-70%, followed by the mitral and aortic (20-30%). More than one valve is involved in 5-10% of cases. Mortality is 5% in tricuspid, and surgery is needed in 2%. In left-sided the mortality is 20-30%, with only a slight impact of surgery. HIV (+) patients respond similarly to treatment, if not severely immunocompromised.
Ref.: Infect Dis Clin North Am 2002; 16: 273-95.

TROPICAL MENACE

Walking past a thick Guyanese canebrake,

She was bitten by a fer-de-lance snake.

A swollen extremity,

Hemoglobin filled her pee.

The family then had to hold a wake.

Note: Two of our residents spent several weeks in a Guyanese hospital on the South American coast. This fatal case of fulminant hemolysis and acute kidney injury from Bothrops atrox toxin was particularly devastating. These are large (3-5 feet long), heavy-bodied pit vipers, which are camouflaged and can strike with high speed and without warning. Among the toxins in the venom are hemolysins. Unless treatment with antivenom within 2 hours is given, a high mortality rate is seen. Other complications are hemorrhage, edema, blistering and necrosis. The major causes of death (10% mortality) are AKI and cerebral bleeding.

Ref.: Toxicon 2002; 40:1107-1114.

A PERFECT STORM

An epidemic that is quite obscene.

Heart disease, lung damage, bad teeth are seen.

Recipes on the internet,

Explosions and fires you will get.

All due to abusing methamphetamine.

Note: I took this title from the reference. Meth is a highly addictive street drug, which is made in "super labs" in the West and Mexico, but can be produced in makeshift home labs from readily available ingredients. These are growing exponentially. Recipes are on the web and can be passed from user to user. The basic ingredients can fit into a suitcase. Rural settings are chosen to hide the chemical smells from neighbors and police. Complications include agitation, mood disorders, violent behavior, mania, psychosis, cardiomyopathy, dysrhythmias, STD's, pulmonary edema, hypertension, dental disease and many others. After explosions and fires, emergency rescue teams are in danger from volatilized chemicals.

Ref.:Mayo Clin Proc 2006; 81:77-84.

TICK TULAREMIA

Young male roofer was bitten by a tick.

Skin ulcer but really was not that sick.

Fever, nodes, leukopenia,

Treated for tularemia.

Late titer nailed a diagnosis quite slick.

Note: Fortunately, this man was working on the roof of one of our residents. The convalescent titer was later drawn on the roof by his brother-in-law, a pediatric ID fellow. Tick tularemia is typically of the ulceroglandular variety. It is much more prevalent west of Old Man River. Arkansas and Missouri have been the leading states for tularemia, with over 50% of cases caused by ticks. In one report of tularemia in Georgia, only 5% involved a tick. To illustrate the "blind spot" of this problem and how physicians avoid genitorectal exams, I will cite a CPC from St. Louis (Am J Med 1984; 77:117-24) where a groin tick was not discovered until the autopsy in a fatal case of tularemia (F. tularensis grows slowly in the lab and can endanger personnel).

Ref: The early Vanderbilt experience: Medicine 1985; 64:251-269.

IMMUNOSUPPRESSION AND HBV

A poorly taught danger of chemotherapy

Is reactivation of hepatitis B.

Patients should be tested before,

Or bad news may be in store.

But there is still a lot of controversy.

Note: Patients starting chemo- or immunosuppressive therapy are at risk of HBV reactivation. A systematic review of 14 studies evaluated 550 HBsAg-positive subjects receiving cancer chemotherapy. HBV reactivation (37%), hepatitis (33%), liver failure (13%), and death (6%) were seen. Prophylactic use of lamivudine was effective in decreasing the risk by 79-100%, but not post hoc. The CDC and NIH recommend testing for HBV prior to giving chemo- or immunosuppressive therapy. AASLD guidelines recommend prophylactic antiviral regimens for patients who are HBsAg-positive in this situation. Rituximab and anti-TNF drugs may be particular culprits.

Refs: Ann Intern Med 2008; 148: 519; 2012; 156:743.

PAINFUL LEG IN A DIALYSIS PATIENT

Getting shots for anemia of dialysis.

Swollen right thigh, could it be thrombosis?

Recent stick blew the plunger back;

Long needle had split the plaque.

Pseudoaneurysm was the diagnosis.

Note: This slender, elderly man was on home hemodialysis in the era before erythropoietin. He was prescribed 200 mg of testosterone IM weekly. This was the only treatment of uremic anemia that was helpful at that time, other than red blood cell transfusions. The latter were only done at very low hematocrits to prevent sensitization to transplant antigens. The history of the plunger of the syringe being propelled backward due to arterial pressure came after the nephrologist delved further into the "DVT" diagnosis. In giving himself the androgen shot IM the patient had hit the femoral artery and created a large pseudoaneurysm. Surgical repair was successful.

Ref: See UpToDate.

TOO MUCH FAT IN THE BLOOD

He was eating ice cream scoop after scoop.

Pancreatitis then threw him for a loop.

Triglycerides high, you might've guessed,

Liver edge at the iliac crest.

His blood looked like cream of tomato soup.

Note: This was his fourth episode of acute pancreatitis. His past history was one of non-compliance with diabetic diet and medications. He ate anything he felt like eating. He was moderately obese and was on no medications for hyperlipidemia either. The serum triglyceride was 5250 mg/dl on arrival. He had fatty liver. There were no eruptive xanthomas. We looked at his retinas later when TG's were better controlled and did not see lipemia there. This is the third leading cause of acute pancreatitis after gall stones and ethanol. Management in this man will involve getting his cooperation with diet and medications. He needs to lose obese weight and control both serum lipids and glucose.

Refs.: J Clin Gastroentrol 2003; 36:54; NEJM 2005; 353:823 and 2004; 350:1235.

ONLY THE GOOD DIE YOUNG

A sudden, unexplained death is brutal.

Pursuing its cause is often futile.

In a Mayo paper that's "arresting",

Post-mortem genetic testing

Provided loved ones with findings quite utile.

Note: In this report titled "Cardiac Channel Molecular Autopsy", 173 consecutive cases of autopsy-negative, sudden unexplained death were evaluated by PCR, HPLC, and DNA sequencing. The average age was 18.4 years, 62% were male and 89% were white. A comprehensive mutational analysis of the long QT syndrome susceptibility genes and a targeted analysis of the catecholaminergic polymorphic ventricular tachycardia type 1 gene were conducted. Overall, 45 putative pathogenic mutations were identified (26%). Females (39%) had a higher yield than males (18%). A positive family history gave a 2-fold higher yield but was often absent. Obviously, we are in the early stages, and more work needs to be done.

Ref.: Mayo Clin Proc 2012; 87:524-39.

ISCHEMIC HEPATOPATHY

It is seen in failing right heart function,

Pericardial tamponade or constriction.

Big increases in AST,

INR and ALT.

Improve cardiac output for correction.

Note: There is decreased hepatic blood flow from low cardiac output and venous congestion with perisinusoidal edema. Both impair oxygenation and lead toward centrilobular necrosis. Zone 3 of the hepatic lobule is most affected. There may be reperfusion damage, too. Dramatic rises in AST and ALT, e.g. into the 5,000's, are misdiagnosed as viral hepatitis. The INR also strikingly rises and is not correctible by vitamin K. Serum albumin values can decrease by 30-50%. Bilirubin is less affected. Effective therapy of right-sided CHF or pericardial disease will rapidly restore order in the lab values. Prolonged congestion (high inferior vena caval pressures) can lead to hepatic fibrosis.

Refs.: Clin Liver Dis 2002; 6:947; Am J Med 2000; 109:109.

MAN WITH HYPERCALCEMIA

Lung and liver granulomatosis,

Given prednisone for "sarcoidosis".

Months later he can't swallow;

Tongue had a colored furrow.

Biopsy revealed histoplasmosis.

Note: Review of the original admission demonstrated non-caseating granulomas in the two tissues and no fungi on modified PAS staining (silver stains were not done). The tongue biopsy during the second admission 3 months later showed numerous small yeasts compatible with Histoplasma capsulatum and one larger yeast with a broad-based bud, typical of blastomycosis. Additionally, the urine histo. antigen test was negative during the first admission. However, a case can be made for this all being disseminated histoplasmosis, with an increasing organism burden from prednisone. The patient was immediately better on itraconazole.

Refs.: Am J Med 1985;78:881-4; Medicine 1980; 59:1-33.

FUNGAL ARTERIAL EMBOLI

Transfusions for marrow fibrosis,

Iron excess causing hemosiderosis.

Skin lesions continued to grow,

Heart valve mass seen on echo.

Iron binder led to mucormycosis.

Note: This was a case of "culture-negative" endocarditis. There was a 1x1x0.9 cm3 lesion on the mitral valve, which was surgically resected. The hyphal mass grew out one of the Mucor group, Cunninghamella bertholletiae. The skin lesions looked liked embolic phenomena and were increasing in number. They were not biopsied. The patient died of cerebral emboli. Non-candidal, fungal endocarditis is notorious for being missed and having negative blood cultures. Ways around this could be a skin biopsy of embolic lesions and drawing arterial blood for culture using fungal media. Deferoxamine (predisposes to mucormycosis) must be avoided in compromised hosts. Newer iron chelators don't do this.

Refs.: Curr Opin Infect Dis 2008; 21:620; Am J Med 1974; 56:506-21.

ABBREVIATIONS

AASLD	American Association for the Study of Liver Diseases
ACEI	angiotensin converting enzyme inhibitor
ADH	antidiuretic hormone (vasopressin)
AIDS	acquired immunodeficiency syndrome
AKI	acute kidney injury
ALT	alanine aminotransferase
AML	acute myelocytic leukemia
ANCA	antineutrophil cytoplasmic antibody
ARB	angiotensin II receptor antagonist
AST	aspartate aminotransferase
BP	blood pressure
BPH	benign prostatic hypertrophy
Bronch	bronchoscopy
BUN	blood urea nitrogen
CC	chief complaint
CDC	Centers for Disease Control
CHF	congestive heart failure
CKD	chronic kidney disease
Cl	chloride
CML	chronic myelocytic leukemia
CMMG	toxic metabolite of acyclovir et al
CNS	central nervous system
COX	cyclooxygenase
CPC	clinicopathologic conference
CT	computed tomography (scan)

D-five	5% dextrose solution
DNA	deoxyribonucleic acid
DVT	deep venous thrombosis
EGD	esophagogastroduodenoscopy
EKG	electrocardiogram
ENAC	renal epithelial sodium channel
ENT	ear, nose and throat
EPO	erythropoietin
ESRD	end-stage renal disease
G-CSF	granulocyte colony-stimulating factor
GERD	gastroesophageal reflux disease
GFR	glomerular filtration rate
GI	gastrointestinal
GM-CSF	granulocyte macrophage colony-stimulating factor
HAART	highly active antiretroviral therapy
HAMP	gene for hepcidin
HBV	hepatitis B
HBsAg	hepatitis B surface antigen
HCV	hepatitis C
HIF	hypoxia-inducible factor
HIV	human immunodeficiency virus
HPLC	high performance liquid chromatography
IBD	inflammatory bowel disease
ICD	implantable cardioverter – defibrillator

ID	infectious diseases
IM	intramuscular
INR	international normalized ratio (coagulation test)
IV	intravenous
IVDA	intravenous drug abuse
K	potassium
Kg	kilogram
LPR	laryngopharyngeal reflux
Meq	milliequivalent
MIP	macrophage inflammatory protein
MM	multiple myeloma
MRSA	methicillin-resistant staphylococcus aureus
Na	sodium
NF-KB	nuclear factor kappa B
NH4CL	ammonium chloride
NIH	National Institutes of Health
NSAID	non-steroidal anti-inflammatory drug
O2	oxygen
OCD	obsessive-compulsive disorder
OR	operating room
OSM	osmolality
PA	posterior-anterior
PAS	a common stain for tissue sections
PCR	polymerase chain reaction test

PEG	polyethylene glycol; percutaneous endoscopic gastrostomy
PIGA	mutated gene causing PNH
PNH	paroxysmal nocturnal hemoglobinuria
PPI	proton pump inhibitor
PTHrp	parathyroid hormone-related peptide
QT	interval between Q and T waves in EKGs
RANKL	receptor activator for NF-KB ligand
SIRS	systemic inflammatory response syndrome
STD	sexually transmitted disease
TEE	transesophageal echocardiogram
TG	triglyceride
TNF	tumor necrosis factor
TTR	transthyretin
UTI	urinary tract infection
US	ultrasound
VA	Veterans Administration

INDEX - MEDICAL LIMERICKS II

A salute to Edwin Newman 28
Acyclovir crystals 74
Acyclovir 73
Addison 17
Adrenal crisis 17
Adrenal insufficiency 17
Alcoholism 27
Allergic reactions to insect stings 57
Allopurinol 6
Amiloride 48
Amyloidoses(hereditary) 26
Amyloidosis (of dialysis) 68
Anemia 86
Anion gap (high anion gap with
  no osmolar gap) 88
Anion gap (normal) metabolic acidosis 91
Antifreeze 65
AST, ALT (high) 50, 101
Atheroembolism 9
Atherosclerosis 9

Back pain 83
Beer potomania 15
Benzocaine 39
Beta 2 M amyloid 68
Biliary T-tube 91
Blastomycosis 102
Blue toes 9
Bowel prep 37
Breast cancer 33
Bronchoscopy 39
BUN/creatinine ratio (increased) 71

C.difficile 80

Calcium oxalate monohydrate ....65 , 88
Carbon monoxide..34
Cardiac channel molecular autopsy 100
Cartoons 53
Cast nephropathy..79
Catheters(arterial) 9
Catheters (hemodialysis) 11
Cavitary lung disease 42
Cell phones..21
Central venous catheters...1
Cerebral aneurysm (banding) 31
Chemotherapy 97
Cholesterol embolism 9
Cirrhosis 32, 84
Clients 64
Clostridium septicum..67
Cocaine contaminated with levamisole.............81, 87
Coccidiomycosis...10
Coca-Cola addiction 90
Colon cancer 67
Compensatory hypertrophy (kidney).....................12
Constrictive pericarditis..7
Consults..75
Creatinine increased but BUN stays
   roughly the same..70
Creatinine (increased) in patient with
   one kidney...69
Crohn's disease...14, 36
Cryoglobulin vasculitis 84
Curvularia keratitis...25
Cyclosporine 40

Daily Weight 16
Deferoxamine..103
Dermatitis hiemalis (winter itch)............................44
Desmopressin 4

Dialysis mortality 11
Dialysis patient (painful leg) 98
"Dirty" urine 49
Diuresis 16
Doctor-patient relationship 64
DVT 98

Edwin Newman 28
EGD 39
Electric home 34
Emphysema on chest films 45
ENAC 46, 48
Endocarditis (culture-negative) 103
Endocarditis 40, 93
Enuresis 4
Eosinophilia 9
EPO 41
Eponyms 3
ESRD (anemia) 86
Ethylene glycol poisoning 65, 88
Excellence in patient care 60
Exophthalmos 77

Febuxostat 6
Fistula First 1
Fleet enema 37
Fournier's gangrene 63
Fungal arterial emboli 103
Fungal keratitis 25

Gas gangrene 67
G-CSF 80
Genital/rectal exams 54, 96
Ginseng lung 42
Glitazones 46

Glomerular hypertrophy 5
Glomerulonephritis 84
Gout 6, 40
Graves (pseudo-Graves) 77
Great disease 22

Head and neck cancer 27
Heart failure 29
Hematuria 66
Hemochromatosis (juvenile) 86
Hemodialysis catheters 11
Hemoglobinuria 94
Hemolysis 94
Hemorrhage 71, 80
Hepatic failure 33
Hepatic fibrosis 101
Hepatitis B 97
Hepatitis C 84
Hepatocellular carcinoma 84
Hepatoerythropoiesis 41
Hepatoma 84
Hepcidin 86
Hip pain (in dialysis patients) 68
Histoplasmosis 102
HIV 10
Human papilloma virus 27
Hymenoptera 57
Hyperaldosteronism (mimics) 48
Hypercalcemia 76, 85, 102
Hyperkalemia 17
Hyperkalemia (drugs) 58
Hypernatremia 31, 59
Hyperparathyroidism (primary) 85
Hypodipsia 31
Hypokalemia 48
Hyponatremia 4, 15, 17, 90

Inflammatory bowel disease 14
ICD (defibrillator) 11
Immune deficiency..10
Immunosuppression and HBV 97
Immunosuppression..10
Infliximab 36
Injection drug use..84
INR rises (not correctible by vitamin K) 101
Interstitial nephritis 35
Intraductal breast carcinoma...33
Iron binder 103
Iron deficiency 18
Ischemic hepatopathy...101
IV drug abuse endocarditis 93

Kidney (compensatory enlargement)....................................12

Language of medicine 28, 49-53, 64, 72
Lanolin..44
Lanthanum (pills seen on X-ray) 89
Laryngopharyngeal reflux...47
Leg pain (in a dialysis patient) 98
Levamisole 87
Liddle syndrome 48
Lithiasis...85
Livedo reticularis 9
Liver failure...33, 101
Liver tumor 86
Long QT syndrome 100
LPR..47
Lung abscess 55
Lung (cavitary lung disease) 42
Lupus nephritis 30
Lyme disease in Tennessee 30
Lymphoma...22

112

Malaria (falciparum) 61
Meningitis 10
Metabolic acidosis (normal anion gap) 91
Metastasis to the eye 77
Methamphetamine 95
Methemoglobinemia 39
Methylene blue 39
Mononucleosis-like illness 7
Moraxella 38
MRSA endocarditis 40
Mucormycosis 103
Multiple myeloma 79, 83
Mycotic aneurysm 93
Myelofibrosis 82
Myeloma kidney 79

Necrosis of lung parenchyma 55
Needle-shaped crystals 74
Neutropenia (drug-induced) 81
Neutrophilia 80
NF-KB 8
Nitrofurantoin lung 56
Nitrogen in diets 71
Normocephalic, atraumatic 51

Obstructive uropathy 69
OCD nephrology 3
Oglala Sioux 29
Oligo-mega-nephronia 5
Oliguria post uninephrectomy 69
Osteitis fibrosa cystica 85
Osteopenia 85

Pacemakers 11
Pancreatitis (from triglyceridemia) 99

Pancytopenia 83
Panhypopituitarism 13
PEG tubes 19
PEG-ylated 19
Pericardial constriction 7
Perirectal abscess 63
Phosphate binder 89
Phosphate (as bowel prep) 37
Pica 18
Plain-spoken 72
Pneumonia 10
PNH 24
Podagra 6
Popliteal artery 93
Primary hyperaldosteronism (mimic) 48
Primary hyperparathyroidism 85
Pseudoaneurysm (in a dialysis patient) 98
Pseudo-nephrotoxicity 70
Pseudotumor mediastinii 78

Raw oyster eaters 32
Reactive oxygen species 8
Rectal examination 54
Refugee 61
Regional enteritis 14
Renal atrophy (unilateral) 12
Renal oxalosis 88
Renal transplant recipients 40
Renal US 69
Rhabdomyolysis 50, 92
Rhythm 52

Sarcoidosis 78, 102
Septicemia (primary) 32

114

Serum urate......6
SIAADH......4
Sickle trait (rhabdomyolysis in exercise)......92
SIRS syndrome......80
Skin ulcer......96
Smoking......23
Snake bite (fer de lance)......94
Sodium urate......6
Solute......15
Spinning......92
Splenomegaly......82
Sporothrix......42
Squamous cell carcinoma......27
St. Thomas Hospital......20
Steroids......10, 71, 80, 102
Strongyloides......2
Subcutaneous emphysema......67
Sudden unexplained death......100
Sun dance......29

TEE......39
Thiazolidinediones......46
Thigh (swollen)......98
Thirst center......31
Three glass or three tube test......66
Thrombotic vasculopathy......87
Tick tularemia......96
Tobacco......23, 27
Tongue (colored furrow)......102
Tophi......6
Transamin......50
Transthyretin (TTR)......26
Triad of excellence......60
Triamterene......48
Trichuris suis......14

Triglycerides (high) 99
Tropical menace (fer-de-lance) 94
T-Tube metabolic acidosis 91
Tularemia 96

Ulcerative colitis 14
Upper esophageal sphincter 47
Urate ("uric acid") 6
Urinary infections (recurrent) 56
Urine osmolality 15, 31

Valacyclovir neurotoxicity 73
Vasculitis 87
Ventricular tachycardia
 (catecholaminergic polymorphic) 100
Vibrio vulnificus 32
Visicol 37

Warfarin 43
Winter itch 44
Wound infections 32

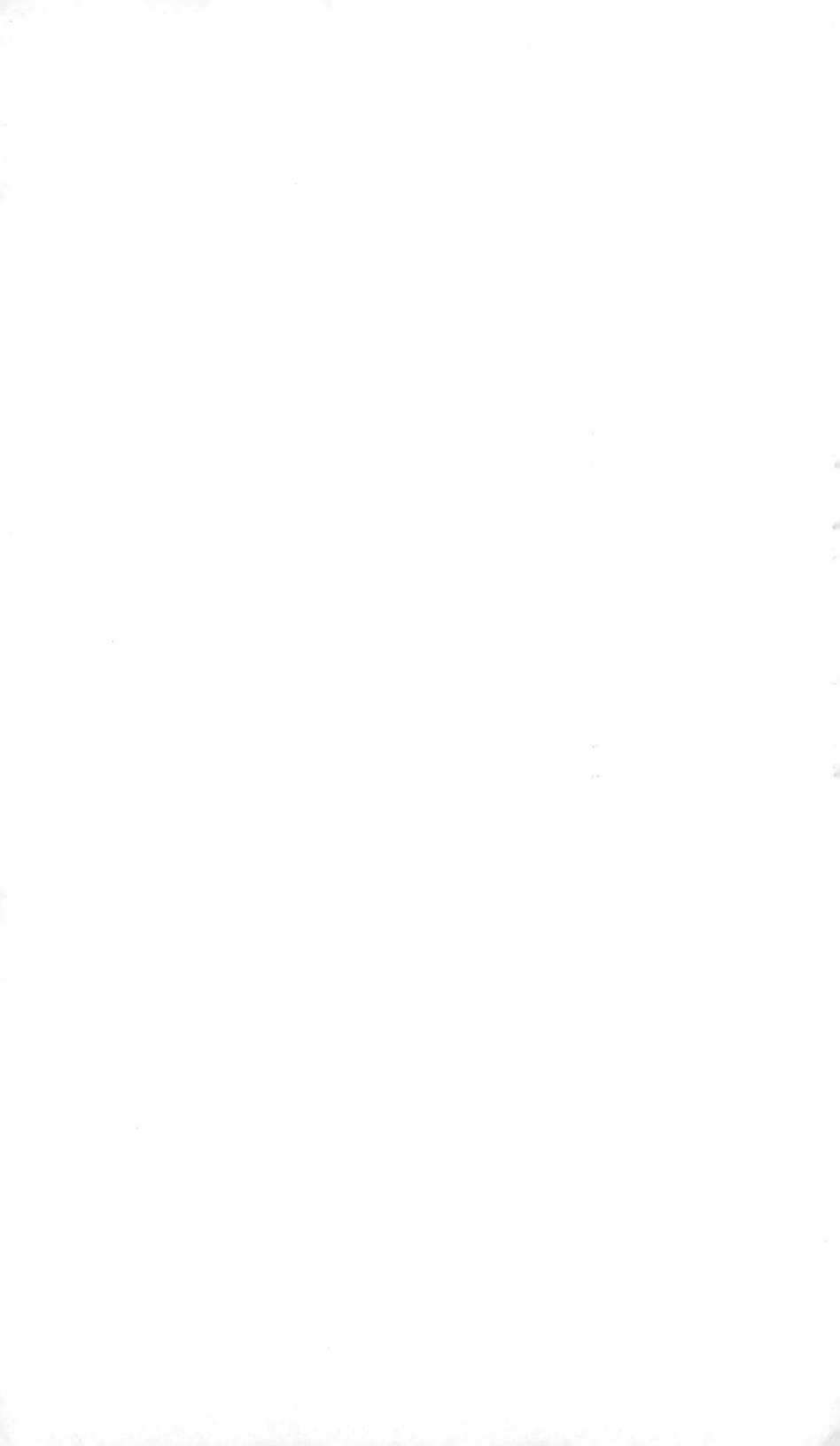

Made in the USA
Middletown, DE
15 June 2016